SLEEP NINJA

®

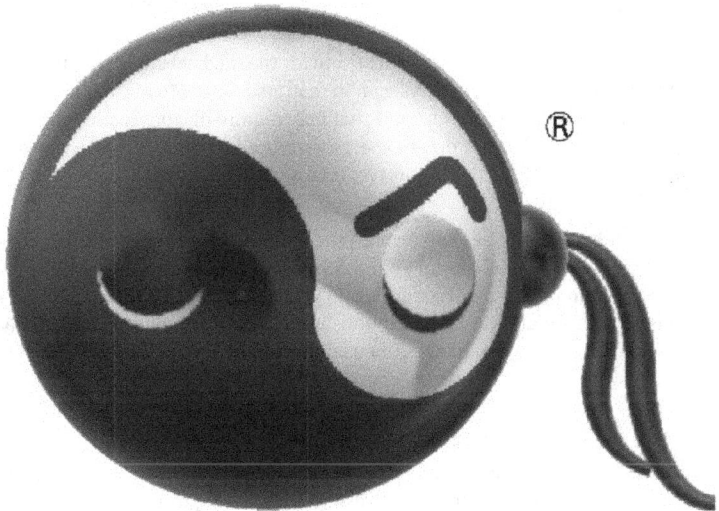

THIS BOOK WILL HELP YOU SLEEP, NOT BECAUSE IT'S BORING BUT BECAUSE IT CONTAINS RELEVANT INFORMATION AND POWERFUL TECHNIQUES!

KARL ROLLISON

This first edition first published in 2019.

Stress / Sleep Ninja Logo is a Registered Trademark.

Cover image & design© Karl Rollison.

Text © Karl Rollison.

Logo Design: Karl Rollison.

Photos and Illustrations: Karl Rollison.

Copyright © Karl Rollison 2019.

This book is not intended as a substitute for the medical advice of physicians. The reader should regularly consult a physician in matters relating to his/her health and particularly with respect to any symptoms that may require diagnosis or medical attention. If professional advice or other expert assistance is required, the service of a competent professional should be sought.

The advice, strategies and techniques contained herein may not be suitable for your specific situation and are for your information and education only. The publisher is not engaged in professional services, and you should consult with a relevant professional where appropriate. Neither the publisher nor author shall be liable for any loss of profit of other commercial or personal damages, including but not limited to special, incidental, consequential, and or other damages.

Any application of the ideas, techniques and suggestions in this publication are at the reader's sole discretion and risk. The author and publisher expressly disclaim responsibility for any adverse effects arising from the readers actions.

The right of Karl Rollison to be identified as the author of this work has been asserted by him in accordance with the Copyright, Design and Patent Act 1988. This is a work of nonfiction but, due to client confidentiality, all names have been changed.

All rights reserved. Without limiting the rights under the copyright reserved above, no part of this publication may be reproduced, stored in, or introduced into a retrieval system, or transmitted in any form or by any means (electronic, mechanical, photocopying, recording, or otherwise) without prior written permission.

For more information regarding Karl Rollison, his products and services visit: karlrollison.com

ISBN 978 1 9164109 1 6

Dedicated to my amazing wife Suzanne who has made this book possible and for offering constant, soft, gentle words of encouragement like...

"Shut your moanie mouth and man up".

Thank you to:

Anne Jirsch and Coner Corderoy for your ongoing professional support.

Thank you to my proof reading / editing team and fantastic friends:

Darren Cherry

Adam Kennard

Lee Velleman

Phil 'Wendy' White

A big thank you to 'Delicate' Dave Willats for your ongoing loyalty and support and by offering simplistic advice in a pointy gruntie, ape-man type way.

Thanks, as always, to the man that set me on this path in the first place, Mr Sean Hackett – a true (and somewhat eccentric) gentleman and proper mate.

...and of course to my beautiful cat 'Alien' for sitting on my shoulders and keeping my neck warm while I write.

CONTENTS

INTRODUCTION   7

1 : REST, HYDRATION& HAPPINESS   17

2 : SLEEPING PILLS   27

3 : PREPARING FOR BED DURING THE DAY   33

4 : THE SLEEP ENVIRONMENT   51

5 : DECLUTTER YOUR MIND   69

6 : THE DETAILS   87

7 : HONEY   97

8 : PREPARING FOR BED AT NIGHT   111

9 : BREATHING   137

10 : QUIETENING THE MIND   153

LAST WORD   167

Introduction

I'd gone to bed at 10pm and dropped off OK but now I was wide awake. I lay there in the pitch darkness with thoughts rushing through my head:

"What am I doing with my life?"

"Where am I heading?"

"Why am I awake?"

"What's going to happen next?"

"How will I cope with the future?"

"I'm going to be exhausted when I get up."

"I wonder how much sleep I'm going to get before I have to face the day?"

This was about the 5th night in a row that I hadn't slept properly. Eventually, the daylight crept into the room and it was time to face the day for real.

So what did 'face the day' actually mean on this occasion? Did I have to shower and put on a suit? Did I need to get in my car and drive to work? Did I have to get a train into the City? Nope. I put on my swimming trunks and walked out onto cool, soft green grass breathing in some of the cleanest, freshest air on the planet. I then strolled onto warm, white sand and slipped into tepid, glass-clear water. I swam for a few minutes and I looked back to take in the view and review my situation.

Think of an island paradise in your mind's eye, chances are it'll be pretty close to what I was looking at. Even though I wasn't too far away I could see the entire island, it was tiny. A collection of mud huts in the middle, a communal/dining area around the edge, all framed with beautiful green foliage and peppered with palm trees with a pale blue, cloudless Fijian sky as the backdrop.

My plan for that day was to have some pancakes for breakfast, some fresh fish cooked in banana leaves for lunch then chill out with a book and an ice-cold beer whilst laying on one of the massive palm tree suspended hammocks. Then later that night, about 10 pm, the island generator would be switched off so the main thing to do would be to go to bed and read a book by the light of a gas lamp.

So why was I having trouble sleeping? I'd just spent a few months in nearby(ish) New Zealand, which is the same time zone, so I wasn't jet lagged...I wasn't stressed was I?

Well, the answer is, yes I was. You see on that island there were no telephones, no mobile phone signals and no Wi-Fi. I was cut off from the world. The only stimulation on the island was conversation, games and books; the simple life. I had no fixed plans and I could have stayed there for months as part of my world tour. I had an open ticket.

This was one of the most remote islands of the 330 that made up the archipelago of Fiji. I planned on staying on this particular island for a month but I only lasted 10 days. I wanted to experience paradise but after a very short period it really wasn't. I was UNDER stimulated; the environmental requirements placed on me were way below my abilities and resources. In other words, I was bored. See one end of the stress scale is burnout and the other end (this situation) is called 'boreout'.

So what's my point about all this? Well, the main reason I was in Fiji in the first place was because I was working in London for the largest bank in the world and at the same time had my own business. It's fair to say I was absolutely, at the sharp end of burnout. When I lay awake at night, not sleeping, I longed for the sanctuary of a far away island in the South Pacific...Be careful what you wish for...

If you're having sleep problems and think that running away to a remote desert island would solve it then think again. I absolutely promise you that for the first few days, weeks or possibly months it WOULD be paradise and you would feel like the master of your environment. I also promise you that, at some point, you would suddenly feel like a caged animal.

Sleep, just like everything else in life, is about balance. When we go on a two week holiday it usually takes about 4 days to unwind from our lives and acclimatise to our new environment. Then most people start to get that feeling of boreout towards the end of the two weeks and are ready to go home. Personally I can't stand two week holidays. That might sound strange from someone who's spent a few years travelling the World but when I travel, as soon as I start to get the feeling of restlessness, I move on to the next place.

Even if you COULD leave your life in search of paradise, take it from one of the few people who have actually done it (on more than one occasion) it doesn't exist. Your perfect life is right under your nose; you just have to manage it better.

So how do I know what I'm talking about? Well, I'm a licensed Harley Street therapist, proficient in a vast cross-section of areas, a registered Hypnotherapist, a qualified life coach, corporate stress management consultant and author of the internationally selling book 'Stress Ninja'. I've also trained in the martial art of

Ninjutsu for 30 years hence the use of the word 'Ninja' in the title of my books.

I've helped people all over the world with every type of sleeping disorder including:

- *Onset insomnia – difficulty falling asleep.*
- *Maintenance insomnia – fall asleep OK but wide awake a few hours later.*
- *Acute insomnia – a short period of disrupted sleep lasting a few months.*
- *Chronic insomnia – a long and sustained period of poor sleep lasting years.*
- *Comorbid – sleep disruption related to a health issue e.g., restless leg syndrome.*

I have experienced most of the above personally. I've always been fascinated with all forms of sleep and I've done a lot of personal experiments with both sleep deprivation and lucid dreaming.

Will this book CURE your insomnia? It might, but I'm not one for elaborate claims and guarantees...However, if you closely follow the information and practise the techniques I PROMISE you it will vastly increase the QUANTITY and QUALITY of your sleep.

CHAPTER 1 :

Rest, Hydration & Happiness

The ultimate goal in life is to be happy. To be happy we need to identify and manage our stress levels. One of the prime mechanisms for reduced stress is to sleep well. Think about ANY situation you could ever find yourself in or have ever found yourself in. There isn't a single situation where being well rested is a disadvantage. It's just so much easier being a human if we have slept well. There is another essential, basic requirement and that's being fully hydrated.

Ok, let me ask you a question:

"What's an example of being tired and dehydrated that you may have experienced?"

I'll tell you, it's a hangover. We all know that being dehydrated causes problems for most of our major organs, especially our brains, but it also affects our hormone production. This directly affects our sleep cycle. Sleeping is a complex series of cycles that are part of our essential daily mental and physical housekeeping and maintenance. Being dehydrated totally disrupts these cycles so even if we have slept, we haven't actually received any of its usual essential benefits.

Remember that most of our body weight is actually water so it makes sense that it plays an essential part in our sleep quality and health, and a lack of it directly leads to the sharp end of stress: anxiety and panic attacks.

There's not much more I can write about hydration other than highlighting two important facts:

1. Forget about the '8 glasses a day' nonsense. This was made up on the spot by two doctors and maintained by (surprise, surprise) the major water companies. In fact, forcing yourself to drink too much water can be very dangerous.

2. We have a very clear and distinct million year old mechanism that lets us know how much water we need and it's called 'thirst'.

This book is about how we can improve our sleep quality and quantity. Sleep really is one of the most important aspects of mental health. What really annoys me is when people almost see it as an inconvenience. I also hate it when people boast about how much sleep they don't need. The reality is that sleep is more relevant in humanity now than it's ever been, yet we are sleeping less than any time in history. On average most people are sleeping 2 hours less than we were 50 years ago. Just look at the statistics for road traffic accidents related to tiredness – they are the highest they've ever been since records began. The occasional night without sleep is bad enough but if it's a continuous issue then this could lead directly to MAJOR health issues including:

- Paranoia

- Disorientation

- Sight problems

- Type 2 diabetes

- Obesity

- Cardiovascular disease

- Strokes

- Depression

- Anxiety

- High blood pressure

- Dementia

- Parkinson's disease

- Digestive issues

People that boast about their sleeping (or lack of) prowess are usually overweight middle aged businessmen who have as many successful businesses as they do ex-wives. The reality is that people like Margaret Thatcher (who only needed 4 hours sleep a night) are few and far between. She had a genetic condition that affects less than 1% of the world's population and it's a defect NOT a superpower. SSS or 'Short Sleeper Syndrome' allows people to function OK on little sleep, but no one escapes the downside of long term insomnia; it has direct links to many forms of dementia, do your own research on the impact of substandard sleep - the sufferers usually acquire some forms of mental deterioration in later life, the sad fact is that you probably know someone who is in this awful situation. Even Margaret Thatcher succumbed to this terrible disease in her later years.

People that try to force themselves to sleep less due to building a business empire are absolute morons in my opinion. I should know because I've been one of those morons...

A few years ago I was coaching an entrepreneur in Dubai who was apparently worth in the region of £50 million.

'You are an extremely successful businessman but you collapse into bed at about 12 then you drag yourself out of it again at around 4 am? So what is it I can help you with?' I asked.

'I just feel anxious, stressed and tired all the time.'

'But you're only sleeping 4 hours a night!'

'That's right,' he beamed. 'I only need 4 hours.'

'But you just told me that you're stressed, anxious and tired all the time. Do you think there is a distinct possibility that perhaps you actually need more than 4 hours sleep?'

'Na, I've always had 4 hours. A lot of people call me the "Machine" because of how hard I

work without rest. Everyone I work with is in awe of my abilities.'

'So let me get this straight: You don't actually need to work and could lie in bed and spend the day relaxing and playing Golf, but instead you choose to work extra hard, mainly to impress people with your prowess, but this regime is actually affecting your health.'

'I don't care. I'm not going to change my sleeping pattern, I'm too busy. There must be other things I can do to deal with the tiredness.'

'You are a highly regarded and well respected, rich, successful powerful business man.'

He slowly nodded with a sly grin, he'd obviously heard this before.

'However, for the record, I don't think you're a machine...I think you're an idiot!'

That wiped the smile of his face.

So just like the 'thirst' mechanism sends us a VERY clear message that it's time to consume liquids we have another powerful mechanism to let us know it's time for 'beddy-byes', it's called 'tiredness' and if you want a happy, healthy life don't ignore it!

CHAPTER 2 :

Sleeping Pills

Ok, so when it comes to sleep remedies we need to maintain an open mind and be prepared to experiment because what works for one person may not be as effective for another. Like most human beings on Earth I have experienced periods of my life where sleep hasn't been as easy as it should and this is when I experiment and play with different potential solutions, I mean after all, none of the stuff in this book is dangerous, toxic or life threatening.

Whatever you do DON'T go down the sleeping tablet route, they are highly addictive and have a plethora of side effects. I'll say this once:

THERE IS NO BENEFIT FROM TAKING PRESCRIBED SLEEPING TABLETS OTHER THAN LINING THE POCKETS OF THE COMPANIES THAT DEVELOPED THEM!

Want more proof? Have you ever taken prescription sleeping tablets? What about over the counter solutions? How about a cold-related sleep aid that promotes 'restful sleep?' I bet you've had personal experience with some, all and possibly others? I'm guessing (as you're reading a book about sleep) that you probably have. Well (honestly now) after taking any sleep remedy have you ever jumped out of bed in the morning feeling refreshed and ready for the rigors of the day? I bet not! They all take a while to fully wake up from and can cause annoying, background fuzziness of concentration that follows you into the morning and even the day. They can even cause EDS or Excessive Daytime Sleepiness.

Years ago I worked on a project with a lovely guy; even though he was young he was very absent minded. I could put up with that, it was the clumsiness that really bothered me, when someone spills coffee over your paperwork, laptop or suit at least once a week it starts to grind on you a bit. He also had mood swings. I really lost my temper with him one day, I'm a reliable, trustworthy, efficient and capable person and this chap was starting to affect my professional image. My theory was that he had an alcohol or drug dependency. He eventually confided in me that he was actually taking quite a heavy dose of prescription sleeping tablets due to his ongoing insomnia. He told me that the irony was that he'd built up a good reputation in his chosen area DESPITE his insomnia and it was actually since he had started on the medication that his performance had declined. He decided to taper off the drugs in a controlled manner. You could actually see the change in him over the weeks. He was a keen photographer and likened the drug reduction period to slowly turning the lens of his digital SLR camera; as the medication and their effects diminished the world around him went from blurry to sharp focus.

Most of this medication has awful physical, mental and emotional side effects including, anxiety, depression, panic attacks and even suicidal tendencies! You are more likely to have an accident, mislay things, have a car crash, underperform at work, have a short temper, get into arguments and have failed relationships. So I ask you, what's the point in having a (fake) regular sleeping pattern if it means existing as a zombie when you are awake? So stick with this book and explore all the chapters in detail and keep coming back to re-read things because you might come across something (or a combination of things) that really resonates with you in particular. After all, when it comes to anything to do with any aspects of mental health and wellbeing, keep one thing in mind:

If it works, it works!

CHAPTER 2 : Sleeping Pills

CHAPTER 3 :

Preparing for bed during the day

What ARE you talking about Karl? How can you prepare for bed in the day!? Well, I'm really talking about making adjustments to your average day in order to more easily *facilitate* the joys of sleep when the day draws to a conclusion.

Caffeine

I love my coffee and I usually stick to one large Latte per day. I have my one and only coffee before 9 am. As with all my writing, I only share stuff that I've tested myself, witnessed or had direct personal feedback. I spent a few weeks whilst writing this book consuming different quantities of caffeine throughout the day. I know everyone is different but, from a personal perspective, if I have just 3 large coffees up to 4pm then I'll still be awake 12 hours later.

This is not just about coffee but anything containing caffeine. Think of caffeine (like alcohol) as a poison which deprives you of sleep and leads to anxiety and panic attacks. Don't be like some of my past clients that have a dependency on high caffeine, high sugar, energy drinks:

"I can't survive without my energy drinks throughout the day because I'm always tired"

Hello! If you didn't drink them in the first place you'd be able to get a good night's sleep, therefore you wouldn't need the awful stuff. This is simple cause and effect.

Alcohol

OK, don't panic, research suggests that a small glass of wine can aid sleep before bed but too much is really bad for our sleep quality. Alcohol is great at dropping us off to sleep but it produces a hormone which doesn't allow sustained sleep. The sleep cycle is disrupted so, although you have been asleep there is little quality sleep, little cell repair, memory filing or general housekeeping that is the whole point of sleep; another contributing factor to hangovers.

Exercise

Just like being well rested and hydrated there isn't ANYTHING on this planet that isn't easier to deal with if we are fit, guess what? That absolutely includes our ability to sleep. Let me tell you what being fit ISN'T, fitness is not having biceps bigger than your head and being able to bench press a small family car. Fitness IS taking your heart to its maximum then, two minutes later it's almost back its resting rate. I've never understood the whole gym thing, you drive to the gym, get changed, workout, shower, change then drive home. That's about 2 hours of your life you'll never see again and for what? To wait around for a sweat-covered piece of equipment only to feel self-conscious because the next person waiting keeps watching you to see when you're going to finish? As a qualified sports performance coach and martial arts instructor, I've helped loads of people get fit but, because I believe simplicity equals efficiency, I like to make things as easy as possible...If you want to get fit in silence then buy some good quality running shoes, open your front door and start running. **It-is-that-simple!**

You don't have to plan it, you don't have to arrange a time, you don't have to stick to a schedule, and you don't have to involve another human being. It's so versatile, you can vary your route, run uphill, downhill, walk, walk-run, jog, sprint, do one mile or a marathon. You can run with someone else, join a club or just go solo. You can measure all aspects of your running from time, distance, elevation, speed, average heart rate, maximum heart rate, and of course recovery rate and you can chose anyone of them to monitor and improve and compete against the only person that you ever need to compete against - yourself. Fitness is all about competing with yourself, competing against others involves ego and ego leads to injury. My ego has assisted me in acquiring a broken nose, broken ribs, broken hands and lots of concussions, suspected fractured skull, chipped teeth and a stab wound to name but a few.

So you can run before you go to work, run to work, run in your lunch break, run home, run after work or run at night (but I wouldn't recommend doing it all in the same day). It's just you and the street. I also love the fact that it's functional, i.e., being able to jog, run or sprint could save your life one day. It's just a personal thing but when we face danger and we experience fight or flight it's usually handy to be able to do at least one of them.

Sorry if I appear biased towards running but, unless you have your own gym or indoor swimming pool, I can't think of a more convenient way of getting fit. Can you?

Sunlight

When we spend a lot of time outside, maybe gardening, having a picnic, having a kick about in the park, going for a long walk or juggling chainsaws on our roof, whatever the outdoor activity is, we usually end up comfortably tired and ready for bed. It was thought for many years that this tiredness was due to excessive fresh air but in actual fact it's mainly down to sunlight. When we are exposed to the sun, even in the winter, our skin produces Vitamin D in response. It's this Vitamin that promotes tiredness and aids a really good night's sleep. I think another contributing factor in the increasing pandemic of stress and sleeplessness is largely due to people spending too much time indoors cuddled up with their technology. This is yet another reason I favour street running as opposed to being in a hot, stuffy gym.

Anyway, my main mission in life is to help as many people as I can to lead a safe, fit, healthy and happy life, so if you are going to spend more time outside you need to remember the importance of using sun cream **NOT JUST** in the summer but all year round. You always have to keep an eye on the future; there's no point in looking a beautiful golden brown throughout your youth only to get that, 'you've got cancer' speech when you're a bit older. Even if you are lucky enough to avoid any skin related health issues from excessive sun exposure, you certainly WON'T escape the wrinkles! So I'd recommend factor 50 all year round but don't just think that's all you need to look for, the SPF (Sun Factor Protection) number only applies to **UVB** protection! You also (and this is what a lot of people don't realise) need to look for the star rating, this ranges from 1 to 5 star and this relates to the **UVA** protection.

Body Clock

There is another relationship between sunlight and our bodies. Our internal body clocks are controlled by how much light we receive but even if we sit inside by a window, or we are in our cars this is still artificial. The truth is that, even though it might seem like our homes and cars are light and bright, they are usually around 100 to a 1000 times darker than actually being outside! The fact is that no amount of artificial light is a substitute for natural daylight and that's exactly what we need for a consistent body clock. The body clock is pretty accurate but is constantly adjusting itself with the use of natural light. The really important time for its first major adjustment is as soon as we wake up. We need to absorb as much light as possible, even if it's dull and overcast outside. We need to look for ways to assist the process. If we go from our home to the car, onto a train then to the office we are not getting any quality light, we should try, for example, to incorporate walking and cycling into our journeys. Try to get outside as much as you can, go for a walk in your lunch break and find excuses to just get out in the open air. If you think of your 'sleep' as a big solar powered battery and every time you get outside, regardless of the weather, you are charging your sleep battery.

Light Therapy

What happens when there isn't enough light to charge your sleep battery? Well there are artificial alternatives. SAD or Seasonal Affected Disorder is a fairly common medical condition and is caused by the naturally lower light levels during the winter months. SAD can lead to a plethora of medical issues and is linked, mainly, to the disrupted production of Melatonin and Serotonin. The solution to this is a light box. I can't tell you any information first hand because I'm quite unusual in the fact that I actually prefer the Winter to the Summer but I have spoken to people who have used them and they seem to be quite effective. Remember though, what works for one person might not work for another.

These Light boxes are surprisingly affordable and worth a punt. You will need to purchase one that is at least 10,000 lux. One lux is equivalent to the light from one candle. This, I believe, qualifies it as a Medical Grade 2 device.

The Flow State

As you can see I'm a big fan of running but it's not just about fitness, it's also my form of meditation. People think that meditation is sitting crossed legged, with your hands on your knees and burning incense, I do that as well but for me running gets me into the flow state a lot quicker.

I started running about 20 years ago and I go through periods of slow half-marathon jogs twice a week to high intensity, one mile, uphill sprints every day. The thing is, every time I start running I hate it, every time! I start off feeling awkward, self conscious, out of breath, my knees hurt and I feel uncoordinated and ungainly. Then, the magic breath happens, I exhale and relax. My running form improves and I suddenly start working as a machine, my breathing slows and, although my technique slows, my speed increases. When this happens my thoughts, worries and anxieties disappear and so does the rest of the world. I go into a trance. This is when I start to have creative ideas. In real terms I've gone into a flow state, I've actually lowered the frequency of my brainwaves. You see, as we rush around in our busy lives our brains are operating from about 30 down to 12 Hertz better known as the 'Beta' state.

When we get into a meditative flow state we are dropping down from around 12 to 7 Hertz. This is the Alpha state; it's the same feeling as daydreaming. I go into more details in my book 'Stress Ninja'.

So try to find your 'thing' that will allow you to reduce the frequency of your brain, it will really assist you at bed time. Think of it as doing a 'soft reset' of your brain whilst you're awake during the day so that when you get to bed you've already got rid of most of the erratic, sleep-preventing, disruptive energy, having done some of the essential housekeeping during the day rather than at night. The fact is, you rarely meet someone who exercises regularly that has problems sleeping.

Daydream Believer

As you saw above we can effectively force a 'reset' but we don't have to. Our millions of years of evolution have developed a perfectly good mechanism for dropping our frequency, it's called 'ultradian rhythm'. Our sleep/wake patterns are called 'circadian rhythms' and they last 24 hours. Now if you think of your sleep /wake cycle as a wave form it should be a nice smooth Sine wave, because that's exactly what it is. Do you think it's a coincidence that we start to feel tired at night and we feel awake in the morning? Nope, our sleep wake cycle is dictated by the circadian rhythm. Throughout the day we are governed by smaller cycles - ultradian rhythms. These go in 90 minute cycles, they are the main reason we daydream and the main reason we have coffee breaks at work and during courses. Think about a course you've been on, they are all about learning, some are relaxed and others are intensive but learning, by its very nature, is very demanding so we can only really concentrate for about 90 minutes.

That's why most courses roughly follow this pattern:

9am registration

10:30 am morning coffee break - 15 min

12:30 - 13:30 lunch

15:00 afternoon coffee break - 15 min

17:30 finish

It's not an accident that most films are an hour and half long. In my book stress ninja I talk about how ignoring these 90 minute cycles can cause massive amounts of stress. This is massively amplified if we ignore the large circadian rhythms. However, if you are drinking coffee and energy drinks to wake you up during the day then having trouble sleeping at night, the wave won't be smooth. We are spiking and crashing. The wave form is erratic. When it comes to smoothing off our daily rhythm, the power is in understanding that we have these 90 minute rhythms. They aren't there to pop up at the most inconvenient times and interfere with our work; they are there to look after us. Have you ever noticed that during a really busy time you'll suddenly start daydreaming? That daydreaming is a wonderful feeling; this is the ultradian rhythm cutting in. So, what do you do about it? Nothing! You don't fight it or panic and you should resist that energy drink that's sitting in your drawer. You just need to go with it and relax. Obviously this requires a bit of common sense, you can't do it if you're responsible for dangerous machinery or other people's lives but recognise that it just a natural system and it will pass. It's your choice if you recognise and go with the natural rhythms and relax or fight against it with caffeine...I call this the 'Ultradian Ultimatum'.

Day Naps

Obviously another way of dropping your brain frequency and resetting your brain throughout the day is via naps. I am a massive fan of Japan, its art, its cars, its culture, its martial arts, its technology, its gardens and of course its (amazing) food! I've been to Japan a few times and one of the things you'll notice is the amount of people that are asleep in public. They're everywhere. On the trains, on park benches, in shops, in cafes, I even saw a Japanese business man asleep in a restaurant. Sleeping in Japan is socially acceptable; some companies even encourage it at work. They have dedicated areas for staff to go and sleep, they call this "inemuri". The important thing is that the period of sleep should be around 20 minutes. Any longer and the sleep is counterproductive, if you sleep too long you will feel groggy and sluggish, if the sleep is too brief it has no effect. This really is a great way to refresh your system and do some housekeeping prior to the main sleep.

The most invigorating and refreshing day naps are done outside (weather permitting), remember the last time you had a snooze outside? Maybe on the beach, by the pool on holiday or just sitting in your garden, remember how wonderful you felt when you woke up?

CHAPTER 4 :

The Sleep Environment

I need to start with a bit of an apology. Sorry if I come across as a bit forceful but I'm a provocative therapist and, when people come to see me for help I don't hold their hands, I tell it as it is. I don't do this for my own ego, or because I'm a bully, I've never bullied anyone in my life. I do this because I genuinely care about everyone and that includes you and I genuinely think sleep is one of THE keys in life to reduced stress and increased happiness.

Our environment really is integral to our security and happiness. Most people are lucky enough to be in a situation where they can control their environment, from little things like adjusting the temperature with a switch to changing the aesthetics with a paintbrush. You may be thinking, so what, doesn't everyone? Well, I want to share a humbling fact with you: over 2 BILLION people in the World don't even have access to fresh, running water. Another fact that shows how messed up things are is that, more people on this planet have access to free Wi-Fi than clean drinking water. Remember that fact next time you're relaxing in a nice deep, hot bath.

If you read my book 'Stress Ninja' then you'll know that there are two states of existence, just two! We are either experiencing growth or we are suffering from protection. Growth is moving forward and protection is moving backwards. Standing still requires no energy expenditure therefore no energy is received in response, this is moving backwards. If you put a human cell in a Petri dish and place toxins on one side and nutrition on the other what do you think would happen? It'll tell you, the cell would move away from the toxin towards the food. This is the same as our environment, if it is in anyway toxic, we will be in protection. Protection is basically our 'fight or flight' response. When we are in protection we produce the stress hormones cortisol and adrenaline. These are not conducive to a good night's sleep.

When it comes to our environment we need to make sure that we monitor it and regularly ask ourselves 'Am I happy here?' Our surrounding areas are constantly changing and these changes have the habit of sneaking up on us. It's a horrible fact of life that working in a fantastic job with lovely people and a great boss doesn't last forever, it can't, people leave and new people start. I've been in a few jobs where jumping out of bed on a Monday morning, looking forward to the week ahead, quickly turned into laying awake on a Sunday night with indigestion and a feeling of dread.

We should ensure that we constantly monitor our environments for potential toxic threats so that we stay happy in the little space we occupy on Earth.

If you work from home you need to ensure that you don't infect your home with work. A dedicated office area is essential, a place where we engage in business, write reports, send emails, make phone calls and when we're finished go back into our home again. Obviously having an actual office in our homes would be ideal but most people don't, so a designated area is sufficient as long as it is stuck to.

I've coached many stressed out professionals over the years, the ones that tell me they can't switch off from work are usually the ones that have infected their homes.

By the same principle we need to take the protection of our bedroom a stage further. We need to make this a place of sleep. Not a cinema, a phone booth, a games room and above all, the most important thing: ***DON'T MAKE IT AN OFFICE.***

Technology

We should consider ridding all of the technology out of our bedrooms; a 'Digital Detox' and that includes the TV and phones. Phones can be charged in the next room so they can't be heard. You're probably thinking, 'What if there's an emergency and someone needs to contact me?' Well, honestly, how many times has that happened in your life? If you have a land line in another room, give the number to the few people that would need to contact you in case of an emergency; this generally isn't a very big list. Alternatively most smart phones can be configured to ring for certain numbers only, even when on silent. This ensures that the phone can be charged outside the bedroom but will still ring from selected numbers. 'Selected Numbers' hopefully means a loved one, not a work colleague or boss. If you're being woken up in the middle of the night with a work issue and it's not part of your original job description, you are not on call, you don't get paid a million pounds a year and you're not a superhero then you seriously need to consider changing jobs!

Alarm Clock

Get an old ticking analogue alarm clock, some people love a ticking clock in their bedroom, I do. If a puppy is having restless nights, a loud ticking clock can be used to calm them down as it reminds them of their mothers heart beat so if it's good enough for dogs it's good enough for me. The other thing about having an alarm clock is to trust it and to stop looking at it...you'll give it a complex. I recommend turning the clock away so you can't see what the time is. I admit that waking up not knowing what the time is takes some getting used to but you also have to have some faith in your own body clock, most of the time you can roughly estimate what the time is. There is something else you can try, waking up without an alarm clock. Make a note of the time then tell yourself out loud the exact time you want to wake up, also try tapping your head with the time. So, for example, if you need to get up at

7am you should say the present time out loud then tell yourself that you wish to wake up at 7am, then tap your head 7 times. This is putting faith in our unconscious minds and setting the 'intention' that we want 'us' to wake 'us' up. The unconscious mind loves it when we firstly, acknowledge its existence then, secondly, put our trust in it. I mean, think about it, alarm clocks have only been around for 300 years but we managed quite well developing the world up to that point without them.

There is definitely a bit of magic about trusting our own body clocks. I think you'll be surprised how well this works but remember what works for one person doesn't necessarily work for another.

If all of this scares you then don't worry, I've helped loads of people sanitise their bedroom and they get used to it very quickly. Remember why we are doing this, so you can sleep better. Can you think of ANYTHING in life that isn't easier if we've had a good night's sleep?

If you are really serious about this sleep thing then you need to take things even further. I'm talking about de-cluttering and redecorating.

Bedroom Floor

There is a lot of opinion that hard flooring is healthier than carpet in the bedroom, I disagree and have my own theories. You see a really important part of having a sleep conducive environment is to have an open window at all times regardless of the weather. This creates a nice airflow. I think that carpets act as filters and grab pollen, dust and other rubbish and keep it localise so it can be picked up by a vacuum cleaner. Hard flooring however doesn't capture anything and allows the dust to perpetually swirl around the bedroom without settling. You will know that I only include stuff that I have tested or can prove, so if you doubt this and you have a hard floor, have a look under your bed, you'll be shocked and disgusted by what you see. A vast sea of dust and hair tumble weeds.

Clutter

OK, so imagine clearing your room and having new, soundproofed underlay and soft deep pile carpet. Then paint the walls in a nice soft tone like an eggshell blue. Remove all the clutter; pack your non-seasonal clothes in vacuum bags and store them somewhere else. Imagine that the lighter the room weighs the better you'll sleep. Think about it from a scientific perspective, everything is comprised of energy and everything vibrates at a quantum level. It therefore makes sense that a room with minimal clutter contains less disruptive energy. Which one would you imagine getting a good quality slumber in, a nice clean, sparse Zen space or being surrounded by piles and piles of dusty clutter?

The Japanese have a word for space. This word is 'ma'. This is quite a hard concept for westerners to understand and as a student of a Japanese martial art for over 30 years I have spent quite a lot of time trying to figure it out, which is quite ironic really because it's not really something you can intellectualise, its more about just 'being'. It's about the importance of the space between objects and the pause between activities. It's about what isn't present rather than what is. Maybe I've got this wrong but what I do know is that, whenever anyone has ever asked me what my favourite thing about Japan is I always respond straight away with 'the Zen gardens'. Tokyo is like a lot of large cities in the world in the sense that it is a sprawling, chaotic, busy, congested, polluted concrete jungle but, unlike other cities, the respite isn't in the form of scattered pockets of well maintained but poorly designed grass and tree littered parks. No, in Tokyo you can suddenly find yourself in the most breathtakingly beautiful spaces on the planet. The emphasis is on the flow of the space. This is the minimalism of Zen. There is peace in space.

The Bed

So let's discuss the bed. The mattress is obviously important but the way I see it, if your mattress is comfortable and you don't wake up with a bad back then why spend thousands on memory foam? Anyway, I know people that have got rid of their expensive newly purchased mattresses because they just don't like them. Not everyone likes a cuddle from their bed, some people like a hard firm surface.

There is an intermediate alternative you can try before you spend thousands; you can buy memory foam mattress tops. These are a few inches thick and simply sit on top of your present mattress and attach to the main mattress with a fitted cover.

The Dark

Another really important thing is to invest in some really good quality black-out blinds or curtains. Let me ask you a question. When was the last time you slept in absolute darkness? Well, most people never do. You see when we were cavemen we had a very distinct sleep cycle (more about that later). There was no artificial light, no street lamps or torches, and hunting in the dark would have resulted in us becoming prey rather than hunting it. But as humans, darkness is needed to promote the production of Melatonin. This hormone is needed to kick-start our sleep cycle. As cavemen there was no light pollution, the night was dense black. There was nothing to do in pitch darkness; there was no entertainment, no reading and no conversation. The dark was a distinct, intense trigger for our bodies to rest. An alternative to blackout blinds are a really good quality eye mask. Don't buy cheap ones like you get free on flights, they don't black out light and rub against the eyelashes which is far from relaxing. You'll need the hard contoured ones that don't touch the eyes or lashes and block out 100% of the light, they form a seal around the eyes and can even help with Hay fever. I would personally recommend the ones produced by a company called 'Bedtime Bliss'. Not only are they highly effective, comfortable and light but they are readily available on Amazon and are great value for money.

You'll know when you have good ones because they will be so light and comfortable you'll forget you're wearing them.

If you wake up in a panic thinking you've gone blind you've probably got a good set.

The Light

OK, so with blackout blinds you can block out natural light but what about the artificial light in your room? Well, I'm a big fan of LED bulbs; they give off more light than their older cousins, emit less heat and are a good deal brighter therefore great for the environment. I have them throughout my property. The problem with them is the same problem found in your phone and table; they emit large amounts of blue light. Our eyes are sensitive to blue light waves which are great during the day but it really is one of the modern enemies of sleep. So if you are going to have LEDs in your bedroom make sure they are dimmable because when you turn them right down they give off a really nice soft glow.

Redesigning your bedroom is the basics. Yes, if you do it properly it will cost you money but how can you put a price on a good night's sleep? It really upsets me that some people almost see sleep as an inconvenience. I also despair when some people are reluctant to spend money on their health, mental health and wellbeing yet they'd quite happily spend thousands on clothes, technology and their cars.

Furniture

Keep furniture to a minimum. Bed side cabinets are really important. It's important to have a glass or bottle of water to hand but it's not so great stepping on them. It's also important to have a light switch or lamp close to hand, some people like to get settled with the light on but it defeats the object if you then need to get up and turn the light off.

So, now you have the basic canvas let's talk about the most important aspect of your environment: **you!**

CHAPTER 4 : The Sleep Environment

CHAPTER 5 :

Declutter your mind

OK now we have a nice clean room, we need to build or rebuild our association with that area. We need to connect the bedroom with sleep and we need to be DISCIPLINED about it.

Have you heard of Pavlovian conditioning? In 1897 Ivan Pavlov, a Russian psychologist published a paper based on his experiments he performed on dogs where he paired food with the audible stimuli of ringing a bell. Eventually the dog would associate the bell ringing with dinnertime. This system is now used throughout the world for training animals. However, it's pretty good for training humans too. We are constantly, subconsciously pairing situations, faces, people and places with all of our senses. We all have songs that remind us of particular occasions or a perfume that reminds us of *that* particular person. The thing is, if you have been spending time in the bedroom with your TV, phone and tablet then you have paired the bedroom environment with stimulation as opposed to relaxation. Now you have cleared the room you can now start to re-associate the bedroom with sleep. This will be easier if the environment looks and feels totally different so you can start with a nice, clean slate.

If we lay in bed with worries running around our minds until we fall asleep chances are we won't have nice pleasant dreams. This is not conducive to quality sleep; I mean after all, have you ever woken up from an intense nightmare feeling refreshed? Probably not. If you're like me, sometimes the nasty dreams and the feelings they promote follow you around all day. So you go to bed feeling anxious, have poor quality sleep and wake up feeling anxious. Is it a surprise that we can fall into the trap of associating the bed and our bedroom to negativity? This is a continuous spiralling cycle and it means that the bedroom (our sanctuary within our sanctuary) becomes a dungeon. I talk more about worry in **chapter 7** but first I want to show you how to break the association with the old bedroom and realign ourselves with the positive energy of the new one?

To help you do this I want you to only go to bed when you are actually tired. Sounds obvious right? But some people go to bed the same time every night regardless of how tired they feel. There are some trains of thought by certain experts that insist that you MUST go to bed at the same time every night. I don't buy into that, I mean, it's a different day with different experiences and you've consumed different food etc. What's the point in lying in bed if you're not tired? That will build up the association of going to bed and not sleeping. ONLY go to bed when you are tired.

What kind of bird are you?

It might seem like a strange question...OK, it **IS** a strange question, but it's actually an extremely relevant one. What I'm actually talking about here is your natural, genetic disposition to sleep, otherwise known as your '**Chronotype**'. There are 3 main categories:

- **Hummingbird.** This category makes up the majority of the population. They wake up at around 7am without too much effort, go to bed around 10:30pm and have a fairly consistent level of alertness throughout the day.

- **Lark.** These people usually wake up before their alarm goes off. They are fully energised in the morning and are those people that are the first person at work looking as fresh as a daisy. However, around late afternoon they begin to run out of steam and are usually asleep on the sofa by 9pm. I know the pattern fairly well because I'm married to one.

- **Owl.** These people need their alarm clock to get them up. They tend to press 'snooze' a lot. They can sleep in till 10am with no problem and need that coffee and morning shower to wake up. They sleep on the train to work. They start to really come to life at night and that's when they have most of their creative ideas. Owls tend to do to bed around midnight. I know this pattern really well because I am one.

It's really important to know what Chronotype you are because it is a genetic thing so why try and fight it? That just causes stress. Like everything else in life, the more you relax into something the better it is. The key thing is IDENTIFYING what bird you are. It really is a case of my favourite quote 'scientia potentia est' or knowledge is power.

There is another thing that I've already hinted at and that's when you and your partner are different bird types, when one is an Owl and the other is a Lark. This can cause all sorts of problems, like 'Why don't you ever go to bed at the same time as me?' Well, now you can explain why. Don't be forced to go to bed at the same time as your partner, in the long run it'll be bad for both of you. I'm not just talking about sleep mismatch causing health issues but it can also put a huge strain on your relationship!

Remember what I said before - **only go to bed when you are tired.**

The bedroom association

Another thing I want you to do is to build up a virtual association to your bed and your bedroom. Wherever you are and whatever you are doing, whenever you feel tired, rather than just sitting there yawning and thinking about grabbing a coffee, I want you to actively imagine walking into your bedroom. I want you to associate into the image (viewing the scene through your own eyes NOT seeing yourself in the image). I want you to associate into the image with ALL your senses. Smell your room, feel the temperature and texture of the floor against your feet. Feel the temperature of the room, breathe in the air. Climb into bed, feel the sheets against your skin.

Another really important thing is that if you find yourself restlessly tossing and turning then don't lay in bed thinking and worrying whilst constantly staring at the alarm clock. Get up and leave the bedroom and go and sit in the lounge and read or write. Resist the urge to pick up your phone or put the TV on.

Don't read, write!

Writing is actually a really powerful thing to do if you can't sleep. Sometimes not being able to sleep is due to worry and anxiety in general life. Writing down worries and observations is what I call 'downloading'. Think of it as clearing space in your brain by giving them a physical presence in the form of words. It's a great opportunity to declutter the brain. Think about it, how often do you sit down in total silence with a pen a pad in your hands and actually write down your thoughts? Here's another thing to think of: there is only one expert on us as an individual, US! Only we know exactly how we feel; only we know what we are thinking. You could be opposite the best team of life coaches and therapists on the planet but they can only go by what you WANT to tell them. You are the only person who is an absolute expert on you. If you sit down in silence and just write, not thinking too much about WHAT you're writing, you might be surprised what comes out. It really is a great thing to do. So there are two ways of writing in order to 'download', consciously and automatic.

1. **Writing consciously**. Actually sit down and ask yourself the following questions:

- Why am I awake?
- What am I worried about?
- What do I need to do to sleep better?
- How can I overcome my issues?
- What do I need to do to achieve my goals?

If you're not in the mood to lament on your life or think about your finances then a really satisfying thing to do is to start writing your bucket list, include countries you'd like to visit, activities you'd like to try, languages or instruments you'd like to learn. Really go into fine detail. If you read my book Stress Ninja you will see in the introduction that writing a bucket list helped drag me out of a bad situation. When I realised that I was in charge of my own destiny, I didn't have to stay stuck; I could do ANYTHING my imagination could come up with.

Yet another thing to write about that is quite enjoyable is to jot down what you'd do if you won the lottery. Ask yourself:

- Who would I help?
- How much would I keep and how much would I give away?
- How many of my friends and family would I take on an exclusive holiday?
- How would I treat myself?
- What type of house would I buy?
- What adventure would I go on?

These questions will kick-start other, more personal and relevant questions to you. Once you start writing it's amazing where things lead to. Exploring your own mind via downloading ideas is a lot healthier and productive then exploring cat videos on YouTube.

2. **Automatic or free writing**. This is where you don't actually have any specific goals or questions for yourself you just need to be relaxed. Get a piece of paper and place the pen on the paper. Then clear your mind and forget that you have a pen in your hand. Focus on your breathing. Breathe in for the count of 5 and really fill your lungs. Pause. Then breathe out for the count of 12, really empty your lungs. You might sit there in a nice quiet relaxed state with an empty sheet of paper. However, you may be surprised to realise that your hand has a life of its own and writing stuff that you have no awareness of. This is a fascinating thing to do and it isn't anything mysterious or scary. It's simply a form of idiomotor response. 'Idio' means idea and 'motor' relates to muscle movement. It's basically a way for the unconscious mind to have a voice.

Don't underestimate this system, I've solved some tricky personal issues and helped many other people using this method. I like to recline in a seated position with a large writing area on my lap, usually a sheet of A3 paper on an A3 clipboard.

Don't underestimate the quiet opportunity to write. It will take you in an amazing direction.

I believe we are happiest when we are creating, be it building a model, sculpting, painting, drawing or even simply cooking . However, this mainly involves equipment and mess, writing doesn't. Want more proof? I wrote 'Stress Ninja' because I went through a period of acute insomnia (sleep difficulties that only last a short period). In my case 6 months. My brain was going at 100 mph every night. However, rather than trying to ignore it I chose to listen to the noise, it felt incredible, I likened it to that little kid in the film 'The Sixth Sense' when he started listening to the ghosts, his problems evaporated. There was a pattern to my thoughts, they were all creative ideas. Once I wrote them all down, I started getting a better night's sleep. I then spent the next few years putting in structure, a framework, adding details and making it flow. Before I knew it I'd produced my first book - Stress Ninja. I've helped lots of people with sleep problems using this precious quiet time to write and there are a few books on Amazon to prove it.

"We are a way for the Cosmos to know itself" – *Carl Sagan*

So let me put this to you: maybe this period of sleeplessness is your nudge to write a book. Going to bed having written another chapter of your book almost compensates for the lack of sleep and when you are tired at work the next day. You would have at least achieved something, rather than having a new list of favourite YouTube videos of skateboarders sliding down stair handrails on their testicles.

As a Hypnotherapist of many years I always find it fascinating that most people have only ever closed their eyes when they want to sleep. Relatively speaking, there are very few people in the world that use self hypnosis or meditation. If there was, the world would be a much better place. On the flip side, most people HAVE to do something when their eyes are open. If you break these programs you will experience some magic.

The dot

So what happens if you find yourself in your front room at 3am and you don't feel like writing? Well, there is a really powerful and simple thing you can try. Get a small piece of masking tape, a label or a section of post-it note and make a small black dot on it. Place it high up on the wall so you can face it whilst sitting in a comfortable position. You need to be aware of the feeling of security and safety. Tell yourself that you want to 'still' your eyes. Then stare at the dot, that's right, just stare. See, the thing is, when our eyes are open they are constantly moving and scanning our environment. This is, amongst other things, for our protection. When we acknowledge that we are safe and we just stare then we are calming the eye movement. Our eyes are linked directly to our brains. When the eyes calm down the mind calms down. It feels wonderful and you'll experience some amazing optical illusions. Because your eyes are not used to being kept still, they will start to feel heavy and you will want to go back to bed.

So can you see what I am getting at with this chapter? Basically, your bedroom should be for sleeping, not thinking, not worrying, not planning, not writing, not reading, not talking, just sleep...well, ok, I know what you are thinking....MAINLY sleep then.

When you practise this you will reprogram your brain to pair the association of the bedroom with the wonderful act of sleep.

CHAPTER 6 :

The Details

OK, so now you have a nice sanitised Zen environment. With little clutter, little furniture, a reduction of 'stuff'. You have also optimised your brain. You have excess thoughts in the night, write them down. You have moments of inspiration, ideas about the future, a shopping list, a bucket list, a wish list, a collection of hopes and dreams? Write them down. There is something very therapeutic about writing stuff down (downloading).

Ok so let's say that you now have a beautiful, new, fresh, shiny, slimmed down, comfy, light and airy, cosy new bedroom. Let's say it's a blank canvas, with lovely deep pile carpet and total black out blinds and a really comfy bed.

You are now able to reprogram your brain to associate the bedroom with sleep. Anything else in your life is done by leaving the bedroom environment. So effectively, you have decluttered your bedroom both physically and mentally.

This is the blank canvas that will allow you to move forward with your sleep program. Now we need to fill in the blanks by paying attention to the details.

The Bedroom Aroma

Natural lavender has been used for 1000s of years to promote and enhance sleep. It has been clinically proven to lower the heart rate, reduce blood pressure and relax muscles. Obviously having a bunch of lavender in the bedroom would be nice but it's not practical so instead buy a really good quality essential oil. I put a small dish on the radiator with essential oil. I also like to spray a high quality lavender spray on the pillows. If you use Lavender enough you will build an association with that lovely smell and feeling tired, your aim should be to tie all of your senses to the bedroom environment. Lavender spray is one little area where spending a few extra pounds will get a good quality item but these products can contain Linalool which is a common allergen, so look out for it on the label. No point in waking up feeling refreshed and ready for the day ahead if your head is the size of a beach ball.

On another serious note, **DO NOT use plug in air fresheners even if they are Lavender scented.** Some of these things contain an artificial cocktail of chemicals, some can even be linked to anxiety. While they may be nice around the home try to keep the bedroom environment high quality, pure and natural.

Sheets

Just like everything else in life, quality speaks for itself. There is nothing better than slipping into clean, fresh sheets, they really do help towards having a great night's sleep. I would suggest buying the best quality, high-grade Egyptian cotton sheets you can afford and aim for a thread count of AT LEAST 200. OK, so they might be twice as expensive as polyester but what price do you put on something that will aid rest? Cotton is breathable and will keep you cool in the summer and warm in the winter, polyester just makes you sweat and sweating causes dehydration which disrupts the essential sleep cycle.

Fresh Air

This is SO important for good sleep. With double and triple glazing now we pretty much live with a fairly low airflow if the windows are closed. Even internal and external doors have insulation and draft exclusion which adds to our homes being hermetically sealed, like living in an artificial, plastic environment. It's only been the last few years that this has been the case. It wasn't that long ago when windows were draughty single panes of glass and doors were low-tech, security devices more about keeping out unwanted guests than fresh air. I think there is a correlation between fresh air and sleep quality. From when we were cavemen right up to the 17th century (when we first started using glass windows) we pretty much slept with the air in our environment being constantly replaced due to poorly designed, gap-riddled apertures. Up until that point, for the previous million odd years since we crawled out of the mud, we breathed nice, clean fresh air when we slept. On the opposite side of things, ever slept in a room that's hot and stuffy with no fresh air? I have, I can tell you, I never jumped out of bed ready for the challenges of the day.

Insect Screens

Some people hate to have the windows open even in the summer. A lot of people allow their irrational fear of bugs and insects to affect the airflow in their bedroom.

Well, I would suggest fitting screens over the window frames. They keep insects out, let fresh air in and also (very importantly) keep Mr Tiddles in. I love sleeping with the windows wide open but it's so much more relaxing knowing that you're not going to be the host of a mosquito banquet and I don't know about you but nothing in this World gets me out of bed quicker than the drone of an angry wasp in the room.

Alarm Clock

OK, as I mentioned in *Chapter 3* you don't have to make your alarm clock feel like you doubt its abilities by looking at it all the time. Turn the clock away so that you can't see the time. When we lower our awareness of time we become less dependent on it. We are telling our unconscious mind that's it's OK to stop making time such a big deal. We become less obsessed with it.

Your Internal Clock

As you also saw in **Chapter 3**, we all carry around a pretty accurate internal clock, this is our circadian rhythm and controlled by a portion of the brain called the hypothalamus. We can use this natural internal clock as an alarm system. When you set your internal alarm you'll be surprised how well it works. It works for me and it works for a lot of people I've showed this to. It may not work for everyone. Once we start to trust our internal clock our subconscious mind will do what it does best: look after us. When we feel looked after we feel secure. When we were cavemen and with our clan we felt protected. When we feel secure and protected we relax. When we relax, we sleep.

Temperature

There is an ideal temperature for a great night sleep and it's a lot lower than you think. Personally I hate sleeping in a warm room. Ever stayed in a hotel where the windows don't open and you didn't know how to (or simply forgot) turn the heating down? You wake up feeling awful, dehydrated with a headache and a dry throat, you then have to pay £10 for a 50 pence bottle of water from the mini-bar. So, how cold should the room be? It's a personal preference but I'd say as cold as you can bear it. I am a bit biased because I actually prefer the winter to the summer! The facts are that the optimum temperature for an ideal night's sleep is between 17 and 19 degrees Celsius (62 and 66 degrees Fahrenheit)

CHAPTER 6 : The Details

CHAPTER 7 :

Honey

So we've discussed hydration and how important water is in aiding quality sleep, I also want to highlight other foodstuffs that are essential for our 'rest quest'. First off though, I want to talk about what to avoid. I want to talk about one of the most sinister substances on the planet; one of the main causes of Alzheimers, Parkinson's disease, brain tumours, anxiety, stress, diabetes and of course, sleeplessness. It is none other than, sweet, innocent SUGAR!

Sugar, Honey & Sleep

We are eating more sugar than at any time in history! Our consumption of it has been skyrocketing year on year for the last three hundred years and we haven't had time to evolve to deal with it. The problem is 'added sugar'. This is stuff added to processed food and drink, not the natural sugars found in fruit and milk etc. Some studies suggest that added sugar consumption has doubled in the last 50 years. Separate UK and US medical research show that Parkinson's, Alzheimer's, diabetes and obesity have also doubled in the last 50 years. Do you see a pattern here? If the end result of adverse sugar consumption is severe, life threatening health issues, doesn't it follow that we will be experiencing massive amounts of stress on the way?

It's no coincidence that STRESSED is DESSERTS spelt backwards.

When we stress we produce Cortisol and Adrenalin. These hormones have a direct effect on our Melatonin production, this affects our sleep. We need sleep in order to grow (there are two states of existence, if we aren't growing we are shrinking) and this is the time when our brains do essential housekeeping, including cell replacement. Like any building work, we need the right materials. It's been proven that when we are tired we crave sugar so we eat rubbish processed food containing sugar.

Did you know that the vast majority of obese people are actually suffering from malnutrition? That's right, these people are consuming excessive quantities of calories all day long but they are actually starving! There is a large amount of stuff going in, but it is not the stuff the body needs. These people are usually unconsciously aware of this. That is why they need to keep eating, because their brains are waiting for the good stuff. I wonder if they fill their cars up with lemonade instead of petrol, hoping that the car doesn't notice.

The brain is in emergency mode so they eat more food to try and stop the cravings, but THIS DOESN'T WORK. So they get fat and then hate their appearance so they comfort eat junk food. In an attempt to control this, they consume diet foods containing sinister artificial sweeteners some of which have been banned in other countries because they have shown to be toxic.

The ironic thing is that saturated fat is actually good for us, we have been eating it since we were cavemen, but fat has been replaced with low fat diet food and drinks containing Trans-fatty Acids, which again are toxins. So not only are we fighting these toxins but the low fat food contains sugar. That's why eating this stuff doesn't satisfy us and actually makes us hungrier, perpetuating this cycle!

WHAT'S THE ANSWER?

SO we all love sweetness. We NEED sugar for energy and to survive. Convenience food is anything but convenient. Diet food is toxic. Diet foods make us hungrier.

Well there IS an answer. There is something that can de-stress us, improve our sleep and, what's more, eating it will actually help us TO LOSE WEIGHT? Too good to be true? This is one time when I believe it IS TRUE. What is this magic potion? Well, it's good old Honey.

Now, I've been promoting honey (unpaid) for many years and I've used it to replace sugar for a long time. There is a little busy coffee shop in Drury Lane that once told me that I account for half the honey they go through in a week. I had a full medical around that time and my blood sugar levels were at the lower side of normal. You know I like to include as much empirical information as possible, so here are the benefits I've experienced myself, and heard from, friends, family and clients, but before I list them: DISCLAIMER TIME.

"If you are planning on changing your diet in any way it is your responsibility to consult your GP."

Get your blood level tested (or purchase an electronic glucose monitor) then weigh yourself each morning. Buy a heart rate monitor and take it a few times a day.

Then what you need to do is buy some good quality set honey. Don't bother with Manuka Honey, it's OK but it's ridiculously expensive and nothing beats the health benefits of locally sourced natural honey. Supermarket honey is OK but it's been through the pasteurisation process. Local honey isn't pasteurised, just filtered therefore the essential enzymes that give it its magical properties are still present.

A full hour before bed, dissolve a tablespoon of honey in hot water. Yes, that's not a typo I said TABLESPOON. Let it dissolve and drink it up.

In the morning, rather than a coffee, dissolve a teaspoonful of honey in hot water. You could put some lemon in with it too. This will kick-start your metabolism and also loads your liver up with glycogen. That's it. After a week or so you will start to notice the difference. You will start to notice an increase in energy, focus and vitality. Go and check your blood levels again. Check your blood pressure and stress gauge readings again. Everything should have come down.

If this is taken seriously the results are amazing. Out of my friends, family and clients I have had reports of:

- High blood sugar levels dropping down to normal in a few weeks
- Borderline diabetics returning to normal in a short time
- Vastly improved sleep patterns
- Massively increased levels of concentration and focus
- Super levels of energy
- Clearer skin and eyes

- Lower blood pressure

- Increase memory

- Vastly reduced aches and pains

- AND, of course, VASTLY reduced levels of stress and anxiety!

I want to share something else with you that you might find hard to comprehend,

This small adjustment will help you lose weight!

Too good to be true? This stuff has absolute magical properties. Read on...

Honey:

- Is one of the ONLY food stuffs that doesn't spoil. Archaeologists have found pots full of honey in Egyptian tombs that dated back over 3000 years, and it was still perfectly edible!

- Is an antioxidant, effectively reducing cell damage.

- Is antibacterial and can be used by vets and doctors to treat wounds.

- Can reduce blood pressure.

- Is an anti-inflammatory, reducing inflammation and swelling, therefore pain.

- Contains antimicrobial properties - kills microorganisms but doesn't harm us.

- Can be an antihistamine, especially local Honey. Great for hay fever, etc.

Excess sugar actually erodes the brain but we have a safety barrier. The problem is, with the barriers up, we can't get fuel and we think we are starving so we crave more high sugar food. OUR BRAINS ARE CONSTANTLY STRESSED.

As you've seen, stress and sleep go together like orange juice and toothpaste.

But here's the really amazing thing:

Honey doesn't trigger the barrier.

The truth is:

We have NEVER in the history of mankind eaten as much sugar as we do now. We have only been eating refined sugar for the past 300 Years. Our bodies don't know how to deal with it. However, we have been eating honey since BEFORE we were human. Our bodies know exactly how to metabolise it! It's like a hug from an old friend. It de-stresses our bodies and our livers, but most of all, our brains!

This means that when we are asleep our brains don't have to stress about how much insulin to produce to store the excess sugar as fat because it knows what to do with honey. It can breathe a sigh of relief. It knows how to use honey and has all the materials to replace cells so we start operating effectively.

I'm not telling you to change your diet. I'm just giving you the facts. Knowledge is Power! However, remember, if you're stressed all the time it's probably because of the GIGO principle, Garbage In equals Garbage Out. If you want to expose yourself to Quality from your environment AND internally, the ONLY result you will get out will be QUALITY. Honey is high in calories but then again it wouldn't be much of an energy food if it wasn't. A quality life has no room for stress! QIQO or Quality In Quality Out.

However, just because honey is good for us and tastes great it doesn't mean we can eat loads of it! Remember, even water is toxic if we consume too much!

There is something else about eating honey that I can personally vouch for, if you include a big dollop in a glass of hot water first thing in the morning it loads up your liver with glycogen, and you don't get a craving for food at all until the late afternoon. I sometimes add honey to high altitude coffee, coconut oil and grass fed butter as well. Butter in coffee? It's gorgeous and gives you great focus and energy. This is my version of 'Bulletproof' coffee, check it out for yourselves.

We can't argue with results. Try the honey diet for a few weeks and see how you feel. It's not chemicals or medication but natural. What have you got to lose? But remember to consult your doctor especially if you have diabetes or any other medical condition.

CHAPTER 8 :

Preparing for bed at night

OK so now you should be lying in a wonderful, clean, harmonious, nice smelling, fresh, technology-detoxed, stress-free area. You have cleansed your mind of distracting thoughts and worries. You are hydrated and your brain has access to clean, comforting, enhancing, amazing, million year old nectar called honey. You are nearly there. Now, you need to PREPARE for bed.

So, as you've seen, the preparation for a good night sleep starts in the day. You can't go through life doing what you want without discipline and expecting to be happy and stress free. You can't go through life, smoking, eating and drinking rubbish expecting a good night's sleep. Sorry, but that's a fact of life. You need balance.

So, you have returned home from work and it's the evening. You have been good all day; you are hydrated and you have avoided excess sugar, alcohol and caffeine but it's not over yet. You have to think about what you're going to have for dinner...

Avoid Refined Carbohydrates

Things like white pasta, cakes, junk food and white bread are high in refined or simple carbohydrates. These inhibit the distribution of serotonin which is necessary to stabilise our moods. Although this hormone is stored throughout the body most of it is actually stored in the stomach. So when we eat well we feel good, this is an example of my concept of QIQO, Quality In Quality Out. When it comes to eating refined carbs I cannot think of a more appropriate example of GIGO, Garbage In Garbage Out, or for a more relevant saying:

Eat bad sleep bad.

Consume simple carbs throughout the whole day and in the evening, when you go to bed you will experience arousal and if you're thinking, 'that sounds great!' then you're thinking about the wrong type of arousal. I'm talking about '***sleep arousal***', this is due to the disruption of melatonin and means that deep sleep (REM – Rapid Eye Movement) is replaced with light sleep (NREM – Non-Rapid Eye Movement) and light sleep is replaced with NO SLEEP.

Discipline

Think about when we treat ourselves to a square of chocolate or one glass of wine. The reward is not just the treat itself but the pat on the back we give ourselves for exercising some discipline. Now think about going back for another square of chocolate but eating the whole bar or going for another glass of wine and finishing the bottle. This can sometimes lead to a feeling of guilt cant it? The thing is we instinctively KNOW what we need to be balanced.

When we feel good through drinking alcohol, eating junk food, sweets/chocolate or taking illicit drugs, that feeling only last for the duration of what we are consuming, we know it's bad but we are putting our short term pleasure first. However, there is a price to pay to, you have to settle the debt with the house, it's not just alcohol that gives us hangovers, we experience a form of hangover from all of the above and they ALL affect our sleep quality.

I'm not in a position to preach to anyone because I go through periods of 'treating myself' but I just love eating salads, veg, fruit, pulses, hydrating and exercise and I can tell you with absolute conviction there is NOTHING in the Universe that makes you feel as good as being fit. When we feel good through healthy choices our bodies operate as

115

machines, we experience 'Homeostasis'. The only price we pay for that is feeling great and amazing sleep quality! This means making the right choices...this requires discipline.

Magnificent Magnesium

I know this guy who told me that his wife was suffering from stress, anxiety and was having trouble sleeping. He hasn't got the greatest attention span so it was pointless me going into too much detail or asking too many questions. I do know that he is a great cook and does all the cooking in his house so I just said to him:

"Search on the internet for foods that contain Magnesium and incorporate as much as you can into her diet". I forgot all about it until a few months later I got accosted on the street but his wife who excitedly told me how good she felt, how well she was sleeping and how shocked she was at how much our diets affect our health. "Why didn't my Doctor tell me about Magnesium? Why does she just palm me off with sleeping tablets?"

The sad fact is that a lot of medical problems can be cured or at least helped with diet, however the sad reality is that most decent body builders know more about nutrition than your average GP. It's not their fault though; Doctors do a great job but don't receive any formal training in nutrition. This is a fairly modern problem because food has been used in all cultures since the beginning of time to deal with health issues.

"Let food be thy medicine, and let medicine be thy food."

- Hippocrates.

Hippocrates is still considered one of the most relevant figures in the history of medicine and is often referred to as the 'father of medicine'. He was born nearly 500 years before Christ and, at a time when life expectancy was very low...

He lived to the age of 90!

Magnesium is actually known as "nature's sedative". It is a muscle relaxant and great at calming the nervous system. It is also the best mineral at reducing stress and anxiety. As I mentioned previously in this book, sleep quality and quantity is at an all time low, one of the reasons is modern farming methods – the magnesium levels in our soil has depleted vastly over the last few years due to modern farming methods and the facts are that most adults have a massive magnesium deficiency. You could reach for the supplements but instead why not just incorporate more natural magnesium into your diet? Luckily, the foods that are rich in magnesium are also some of the nicest. They include:

Fruit - bananas and avocados

Legumes - seeds, chick peas, kidney beans

Nuts – almonds, peanuts, Brazil nuts

Veg – broccoli, peas, cabbage, spinach, asparagus, kale

Fish - Salmon and tuna

A lot of the above food also contains tryptophan. This is an amino acid that, when eaten, produces serotonin in the brain. Serotonin is a mood stabilising neurotransmitter that makes us feel great and promotes sleep. Apparently the best natural source of tryptophan is found in turkey (the bird not the country).

Magnesium Massage

OK, so maybe you're a REALLY fussy eater and you don't like anything on the above menu? Perhaps, you do a lot of exercise and your muscles ache a lot? Maybe you just have general aches and pains? Well magnesium can also be ingested transdermally (through the skin) and there are loads of products on the market that facilitate this. There are:

Body oils

Moisturisers

Shower gels

Makeup

Body sprays

Saving the best for last (and the one that makes the most sense) magnesium bath salts. Which can be used in a...

Hot Bath

For those of us that don't own a bath, a hot shower is nearly as good, the important thing is to be in it for long enough to raise our temperature. When we naturally set about the process of sleep, one of the things that happens is that our body temperature drops. That's why it's so important to keep someone awake if they are suffering from hypothermia, they already have a dangerously low body temperature so falling asleep is fatal. If we have a hot shower or bath we have raised our body temperature. As soon as we get out and dry off our body temperature starts to drop. This fools our bodies into thinking its sleep time.

Temperature

Talking of temperature, as previously mentioned, the room needs to be cool, not just to assist us in falling asleep but actually STAYING asleep. I mean, think about sleeping in a heat wave, if and when we do fall asleep we usually wake up throughout the night. So how cold does the room need to be? A lot colder than you think, research has shown that the optimum temperature of your bedroom should be around 17 to 19 degrees Celsius (approx. 62 to 66 degrees Fahrenheit). I know I've repeated myself but that's because it's a really important and simple aspect of sleep but one that some people are reluctant to adhere to.

Rose Tinted Glasses

Ok, not so much rose tinted as orange, they are actually called 'blue light blockers'. You should put these on in the evening as soon as it's convenient. They block out all forms of blue light and can prevent the very real and increasing CVS or Computer Vision Syndrome. This is a situation caused by staring at screens (all forms of screens) for long period of times. It causes lots of physical problems including vision defects, which in turn lead to sleep disruption which then causes physiological problems. You can purchase a good pair online. The ones with the orange lenses are good but a really important thing is that they are the wraparound type so that they block blue light coming in from the side of your eyes. I know it's not cool to wear sunglasses indoors and you might look a bit like that some idiot rock star but if it assists in a good night's sleep who cares? A really important thing to do is not to allow any light in when you take them off, so you either close your eyes to put on your eye mask or you take them off in the pitch darkness of your bedroom.

Lowering Your Frequency

I spoke about lowering the frequency of your brain in **Chapter 3**. This was, amongst other things, about de-stressing throughout the day and processing stuff that would otherwise be left to bedtime. The thing is we can actually lower the frequency of our brains at anytime. What amazes me is that this is one of the most powerful things we can do to change our mood and mindset yet not many people actually know about it. Here's a basic overview:

Name	Frequency	Use
Beta	12-30 Hertz	This is the usual waking state of being. We experience this at work and when solving problems. You may be in this state right now, but it's not good to stay at this frequency for too long. If you follow the technique in this chapter, you won't be.

Name	Frequency	Use
Alpha	7-12 Hertz	This is being awake but in a relaxed state of mind. This is the frequency we experience when we find ourselves daydreaming
Theta	4 -7 Hertz	This is a state of deep relaxation. This state can be accessed with good deep hypnosis or meditation. We can access this frequency by practising the technique in this chapter
Delta	0.5-4 Hertz	This is the slowest frequency that our brains can operate at. It is when we are in a deep, dreamless sleep. This can be accessed with meditation but usually requires years of training.

If we are walking around in a beta state and we can actually CHOOSE to lower it, what better time to do this than just before bed?

My take on Mindfulness

Sit somewhere soft and comfortable like your sofa and allow yourself to get comfortable. Don't cross your arms or legs. Lower the light level if you can.

Now take a really deep breath in for the count of 5 and breathe out long and slow for the count of 12 until your lungs are completely empty. Notice the pause between the breaths. Repeat. Do this for as many times as you can without feeling dizzy.

Now look around the room and allow your eyes to find something, whatever it is, just allow your eyes to find an object. When you find an object imagine that just looking at it adds weight to your eyelids. Try not to blink.

Keep the awareness of what your breathing is doing. Now just stare at the object and try to imagine what you would look like if you could see yourself from that object. Allow your jaw to relax and I want you to be aware of all the noises in the room, outside the room, in the street outside.

You thoughts will probably wander around. Don't wrestle with the thoughts just observe them and let them flow. Notice the pause between your breaths.

I want you to feel yourself sinking into the chair. See yourself from the object again. Imagine you can see yourself slowly disappearing into the sofa. Become aware of the stinging of your eyes as they get heavier. Have a yawn and allow yourself to relax a bit more. Try in vain to keep your eyelids open.

When you start to feel that lovely drifting sensation of tiredness, get up and drift into bed.

Preparing for bed - The hour before....

Bach (TM) Flower

There are many different types of Bach flower products. I give away boxes of Rescue Remedy chewing gum to certain clients. Some people prefer the spray. This stuff is a safe and gentle way of just quieting the mind and levelling off the body's energy. I quite like the 'Melts', they are tiny capsules that are placed on the tongue, and dissolve instantly allowing the mind to quieten. Rescue Remedy products get good reviews but do your own research. The thing is, this stuff is 100% natural, pretty good value and readily available so what have you got to lose?

Honey

Ok so I've explained the benefits of Honey and, as I said, that can be dissolved in hot water and consumed an hour before bed. It doesn't just have to be in hot water though; you might not like the taste of Honey on its own. You can add it to other sleep-enhancing substances. When added to, for example, tea or coffee it's pretty indistinguishable from sugar. But as you've seen, it's infinitely better for you.

Chamomile Tea

Chamomile tea has been used for centuries dating back to ancient Egypt. It is known for its muscle relaxing and stress relieving properties. It's a pretty amazing combination if you add this to the wonderful soothing properties of Honey.

Cherries and Ginger

These are great natural sources of Melatonin. This is the prime hormone responsible for assisting our natural circadian rhythm.

Brazil nuts

These contain Selenium, which effectively balances out the thyroid. Thyroid imbalance causes restless sleep. As previously mentioned, the more in balance we are, the more we are in homeostasis. This leads to quality sleep.

Walnuts

Walnuts are another great source of tryptophan but you probably won't fancy bunging a turkey in the oven before bed so a handful of walnuts are a handy alternative.

Kiwi fruit

Kiwi fruit is high in serotonin but there is something else that it contains; they are one of the best natural forms of antioxidants on earth. Clinical trials are showing an increasing link between antioxidants and sleep. In case you didn't know, antioxidants basically protect your cells from damage. This just adds to the theory that the more aligned and balanced your whole system is, the better the quality AND quantity of sleep.

Almond Milk

Hot cow's milk has been used for centuries to aid sleep. It contains two ingredients that you now know are beneficial for sleep and relaxation: the hormone melatonin and the amino acid tryptophan. However, Almond milk also contains these ingredients and, although it isn't as nutritious as cow's milk, it does contain Vitamin D which cow's milk doesn't. Also (most importantly) almond milk is fine for people who are lactose intolerant, the symptoms of which, like any allergy, range from mild to severe. The thing is, if you are lactose intolerant, drinking cow's milk before bed certainly won't equate to a good night's sleep. The other thing is - how do you know if you have a mild intolerance or not? Maybe that could be a cause of your disrupted sleep pattern? Anyway, almond milk is readily available, cheap and it tastes great so you may as well give it a bash! One thing to keep an eye on though, is the actual almond content, you obviously want as high a percentage as possible, I personally wouldn't bother with stuff that contains 2%.

Karl's Sleepy Shaky Shake

OK, so this is my own recipe. It hasn't gone through any clinical trials or anything but I have applied my fairly good logic (and intellect) and my instincts have given it the OK. It tastes great and you can do your own version using all the items listed in this chapter but I would avoid using fish if I were you. Anyway, unless you are allergic to any of the ingredients in my Sleep Shake it's hardly going to kill you is it?

Ingredients (serves 2):

5 grams of fresh root ginger (cut the skin off)

10 grams of dried cherries

10 grams or a small handful of almonds

10 grams or a small handful of walnuts

10 grams or a small handful of Brazil nuts

One Chamomile teabag

150 ml (or a cup) of boiling water

Tablespoon of local honey

Two Kiwi fruits

200 ml (a small mug) of unsweetened almond milk

Method:

Place the chamomile teabag in the boiling water and leave for a few minutes.

Put the cherries, nuts, ginger and almond milk in a blender with the honey.

Bruise the Kiwi fruits by rolling them forcefully on your kitchen top. When they have softened cut them in half and squeeze the contents into the blender, discard the skins. Add the Chamomile tea.

Blitz it all up then transfer the liquid into 2 mugs for you and your partner. Alternatively, place half the liquid in the fridge for the following night. You could, of course, drink the whole lot to yourself but you'd need a large mug and you might wake up in the middle of the night for a toilet break which sort of defeats the objective.

Pop the shake in the microwave for 30 seconds.

I love the taste of this because it has a nutty, gingery flavour but it tastes just as good with added powered cinnamon or coco but play around with it until you're happy.

I've made this shake for loads of family and friends. I was going to provide a few case studies and testimonials but, you know what? Just try it for yourself...the proof, as they say, of the pudding is in the eating (pudding in this instance being a sleep shake). I think you're going to be pleasantly surprised.

CHAPTER 9 :

Breathing

I have studied breathing in all its forms since I was a boy - in different martial arts, boxing, meditation and self hypnosis. I have played around with the power of breathing, maybe it was because I know first-hand what it's like to not be able to breathe. When I was a boy my airway closed off, I was rushed to hospital and I nearly died. I haven't taken breathing for granted since. It's funny that most people don't practise any form of breathing manipulation and the only time they think about breathing is when they have difficulty doing it. If you get it right the power of the breath is incredible. Many years ago, whilst touring around Bali I spent a lot of time researching underwater meditation and I managed to stay underwater in a complete trance state for over 3 (supervised) minutes...Don't try that at home! With the help of breathing I've helped people manage pain, achieve super levels of focus, wake up and fall asleep. I've also assisted people in achieving amazing physical feats, including assisting an old lady to tick off an item on her Bucket list of, wait for it, breaking a plank of wood with her bare hands.

Don't underestimate the importance of breathing, it is the basis of every human endeavour; we can create and destroy with our breathing.

Breathing is THE most powerful thing we possess. So, on that basis, why wouldn't it also be the most powerful aid in sleep? Well, it is. The following is a proven technique to promote sleep. You can do your own research but all I can tell you is that I've had great results and feedback using it. The thing I love about it is that it's free, it's totally safe, non toxic and non addictive so what have you go to lose?

Sleep aid. 4-7-8 breathing

Get comfortable in a quiet place and position your tongue on the roof of your mouth behind your teeth.

1. Breathe in deeply through your nose for the count of 4

2. Pause for the count of 7

3. Breathe out for the count of 8 making an 'ahhh' noise as you do this, be aware of your muscles relaxing.

4. Go back to number 1. Keep doing this for as long as possible.

You will, at some point feel a comfortable shift in your energy and anxiety levels

There is another breathing technique I'd like to share with you. This can be done at anytime to allow you to relax. It's really nice to do when you get home from work, you could even do it at work, if you can find a nice quiet area. If not, there's nothing stopping you going for a walk and finding a suitable place outside.

5/12 breathing technique

Sit in a quiet place where you can fully relax. Sit with your back straight.

Close your eyes and place your hands on either side of your stomach just under your ribs.

Keeping your eyes closed gently look up as though looking at the inside of your eyebrows.

Breathe in through your mouth and at the same time imagine that you are breathing in through the back of your hands. This invites the abdomen and diaphragm to the party.

Breathe in deep and fill the lungs from top to bottom. Breathe in for the count of 5.

Pay attention to the pause between breaths.

Purse your lips and imagine you are trying to blow out a candle over the other side of the room. Breathe out of your mouth for the count of 12 or until your lungs are completely empty. If you do this right you will be aware of your stomach sucking in.

Repeat this as many times as you can but stop if you get dizzy.

Hopefully it's clear that sleeping is one of the most important things in our lives and if we are really serious about improving the quality and quantity of our sleep we need to take it really seriously. It isn't a matter of doing one thing, eating one thing or making one change it's a combination of lots of changes. It should also be clear that we need to start the preparation for sleep during the day and there is a physiological process that governs our brain's down-time. Our main rest is controlled by the circadian rhythm and the smaller rests throughout the day by the ultradiun rhythm, the large one goes in 24 hour cycles and the smaller one repeats in 90 minute cycles. We need to protect these rhythms from excessive caffeine and sugar.

Sometimes we need a boost, a 'pick-me-up'. We can do this via a little wake up technique:

WAKE UP - Alternate Nasal breathing

I was first shown this by a Yoga expert in Ubud, Bali, Indonesia - consistently a top destination for Yoga exponents around the globe. It's a form of Pranayama or breath control. As I understand it, it realigns the energies in our bodies and brings the left and right hemispheres of the brain into alignment. It also de-stresses and revitalises. Some of my clients have reduced, or even given up, caffeine by using this method. *REMEMBER, as with any breathing exercise, stop if you get dizzy.*

Cover your right nostril with your right thumb, keep the other finger straight and out of the way, to not restrict the airflow. Take a deep, long breath in. Pause.

Cover your left nostril with your left thumb, fingers up, and breathe out fully through your right nostril. Pause. Then cover your right nostril again and breathe in through your left nostril as before. Keep this cycle of left and right going. Try 10 times on each nostril. You should be aware of a shift in your energy levels, like a caffeine rush.

The waking-up trigger

My initial intention was to write a whole chapter about waking up but I wanted to focus more on the sleep state. I mean waking up for most people is fairly easy especially if you are a 'Lark Chronotype'. My wife Suzanne and I went around the world together and, no matter what situation we were in, how long we had travelled for or what country we were in she would leap out of bed, clap her hands together and say (every single morning):

"Come on Karl, up and at 'em!"

Needless to say this is now one of my least favourite sayings of all time.

Even if you are a 'Hummingbird Chronotype' you are probably fine with getting up. However, for us 'Owl Chronotypes' it's a different story. I can lie in bed all day if I chose to, this is not a medical problem; I can be really good at sleeping if I put my mind to it and I REALLY struggle getting up in the morning. Why am I telling you this? Because most of my career has involved working with City traders therefore most of my professional life required me being *at my desk* in London by 7am without fail. The thing is I try to never be late for anything, I just hate it and being late for work during my time working for Investment banks just wasn't an option so I made myself an expert at waking up. Here's how:

Firing up the Sympathetic nervous system

As soon as your alarm goes off, switch it off. No snooze, no matter how tired you feel!

Then don't climb out of bed, jump out of bed with some energy and vigour. (This is why it's important to put your glass of water on your bed side table and not the floor). As you jump out of bed I want you to SHOUT a power word or statement that gets you fired up (or you could just clap your hands), the important thing is to make a noise. Do something that gives you a positive **punch** of energy.

Turn your light on and stare at it with your eyes as wide as possible, you want as much light getting into your eyes as possible.

You then want to take in 3 really deep breaths. Imagine you are about to swim a length of a swimming pool under water. Like the 5/12 technique above but with a bit more intensity ensuring you don't get dizzy. This is actually powering up your Sympathetic Nervous system which controls the fight or flight response. You are oxygenating your blood and generating adrenaline.

Open the curtains then make your bed as neatly and as quickly as possible. Why? Because you are showing respect and appreciation to your sleeping area (billions of people don't own a bed) and because you haven't even left your room yet but you have already achieved two things:

1. You have woken up on time.

2. You have neatly made your bed with gratitude.

You are setting a precedent of having a productive day.

All of the above, with practice, will become second nature. It usually takes, on average, 60 repetitions of something to form a habit so after a few months you'll be doing this without any effort. We are actually telling our unconscious minds that we are serious about starting our day and getting things done. We are also pairing our chosen power word and statement with waking up. Guess what the side effect of this is? It actually helps reduce procrastination!..

I was going to write a whole chapter on procrastination but I'll do it later...

I used to have 3 alarm clocks, one battery powered analogue, one windup, and one plug-in red LED digital. When an alarm went off, no matter how I felt, how tired or hung-over, I would do the above religiously. My chosen power statement was, "***No option!***". This was because if I never jumped out of bed I would have laid there continuously pressing the snooze button. On the rare occasion I did this I would find myself rushing about in a state of panic. Pressing snooze and having another 9 minutes sleep was bliss but it comes nowhere near the feeling of dread and despair that accompanies the anxiety of missing my train and being late so I literally had *no option* other than getting up. It also referred to the fact that I was brought up on council estates, I was one of the poorest kids in one of the roughest schools in the area and I couldn't read until I was 8 so it also meant that being complacent about having a great career was *no option!*

By the way, don't worry if your waking-up trigger statement is a bit weird. I taught this technique to one of my mates (a fellow Owl) and his trigger statement is:

> *"I want your clothes, your boots and your motorcycle!"* shouted in a bad Arnold Schwarzenegger accent every morning...Imagine what his neighbours must think!?

Hopefully you can see what I'm getting at with all of this stuff. We need to make our sleep / wake cycle as separate, defined and distinct as possible. This will make it a digital, binary process:

"I feel tired; I need to go to bed"

"I'm awake; I need to get away from my bed NOW!"

These clear distinctions are like sitting on a swing. You need to put effort into the forward and back motion before it moves as a smooth pendulum. This gives it a nice smooth rhythm. Everything works better with a smooth, distinct rhythm: the tides, the seasons, the planet, flowers, insects, the universe and, of course, us. We are made up of cycles and rhythms so doesn't it make sense that we get in sync with them rather than fighting against them?

There'll be only one casualty in that war if we don't!

CHAPTER 9 : Breathing

CHAPTER 10 :

Quietening the mind

Quite a common thing that interferes with sleep is the little entity in our heads - the bringer of doom. It tells us little stories and even presents us with images to really build a picture for us. You know the sort of thing, you're cuddled up to your partner and just about to drop off into a wonderful sleep when your brain suggests that you left the oven on. You are slowly presented with visions of jumping out of the window, then the voice pipes up; 'Sarah would never jump out of the window, she hates heights! We'll have to go for the front door, but that means going past the kitchen. Maybe if I throw enough pillows and cushions out of the window and landed on them I could get away without breaking my legs. Damn! My phone's charging in the kitchen. I'll go next door and wake up Terry and borrow his ladder and come back for Sarah. Oh no! He's on holiday and what about the cat? Maybe I better get up and check, just in case!"

The oven is, of course off...so what happened here then? Well, this is what I call the S.T.O.P. or the Stupid Traumatising Over-protective Parent. We all have a little voice in our heads and it's there for our protection. The problem is it tries too hard. You might be thinking that you're not familiar with the concept of S.T.O.P. well that's because it's my own creation so to give it its more common name...***worry***.

If you've read my book 'Stress Ninja', you will already be familiar with the following but I love sharing this because it really does seem to help people put worries and anxiety into context:

> *Take 100 people in any part of the world with a mixture of worries (I'm talking about everyday issues here not terminal illness or death). Imagine these people biting their nails and lying*

awake at night. Now, out of these 100 people 88 of them will never encounter their worry. It just never materialised. Out of the 12 people that did meet their woes 9 people said it wasn't anywhere near as bad as they thought it would be. Of the remaining 3 people 2 said that they wouldn't have changed anything because it was such a great lesson.

'Remember, we learn more from one disaster than from a thousand successes!'

– Karl Rollison

So, anyway, out of the 1 person in 100 who said that the situation they feared was as bad as they thought it would be, in retrospect, all admitted that not only was it a great lesson but it made a great story to tell others.

Mark Twain summed up worry better than anyone, ever:

'I've had a lot of worry in my life, most of which never happened.'

I developed a system years ago that came from teaching women's self defence classes, like most of my stuff it mixes elements of martial arts with hypnosis. Also, like most of my stuff it's very simple. Basically I want you to continue going about your life as you do but I want you to realise that you have access to an awesome security guard: your unconscious mind. Not your conscious mind, your UNCONSCIOUS mind. How do you do this? You've already done it thousands of times in your life, you just didn't realise it. Remember that time where your unconscious mind told you not to take that shortcut, not to get into that car, not to take that job, not to click on the link in that email? Well, the problem is that your conscious mind can override the unconscious, usually with a negative outcome. You know, the feeling after the event when you're angry with yourself and you say something like 'I KNEW I shouldn't have done that!" or "Why didn't I trust my instincts?" or "I had a bad feeling from the start".

Well, call it what you want, a hunch, instinct, intuition, spider sense, god, your guardian angel, 'The Force', it doesn't matter, you know when it occurs and you know what it feels like. Now here's the key thing, summed up by one of the many original quotes that I have created:

REAL instinct, the really important stuff, isn't a little voice, it's a feeling!

Instincts are VERY powerful but people mainly only ever tune into them when it comes to large important things like our safety and life or death decisions. The thing is, these feeling can be tuned into, amplified and applied to our everyday lives.

So think about the last time your instincts announced themselves. How did it feel? Where was that feeling?

For me personally, my instincts are in my stomach. When I consult them if the answer is a negative and that I need to be cautious about a situation then I will get a cold, sinking feeling in the base of my stomach. If however, the situation is all OK then I get a warm feeling that starts at my stomach and travels up to my face. I've helped hundreds of my clients and martial arts students tune into their instincts and everyone has slightly different experiences of how their intuition expresses itself. Just like my 'Stress Meter' concept (which is allows us to monitor our own stress levels) the key thing is to calibrate and tune into your own body. Let me tell you something else too, when people clear out the junk in their heads and stop listening to their S.T.O.P. they ALWAYS go onto great things. I know this because EVERYTHING I do in my life is based on my instincts.

So, in the scenario above, if you are laying in your bed and are worried about whether you have left the oven on, turn down the little voice, go quiet inside and then ask yourself, slowly and deliberately; 'Did – I - switch - the - oven - off?'. You are waiting for your feeling in response NOT a voice or image, a FEELING. Tuning in requires trust. You really need to TRUST your feelings because here's another fact:

If you really tune in and TRUST your feelings they will NEVER let you down.

Again, I know this because mine have NEVER let me down.

The next time you are lying in bed acting out every possible outcome of your life just slow down, relax and ask your instincts whether you really need to spend your time making up fantastic outcomes for a mundane, run-of-the-mill situation. I think you'll be amazed how often your instincts will tell you,

"Everything is absolutely fine and dandy!"

It's a funny situation that we can choose what we spend our time thinking about. We can hope and pray about all the possible great things that could happen to us but instead we focus on the negatives, worry is sort of like reverse praying.

OK, so how do you turn off the S.T.O.P? How do you turn down the little voices of doom in order to tune into your instincts? Well, the most powerful technique I've ever come across is the 'shhh' technique.

STOP the S.T.O.P. – the 'Shhh' technique

The 'shhh' noise is very powerful. Try this, next time you are in a noisy room and you want to get everyone's attention. Rather than trying to shout over the noise, simply make a long 'shhh' noise. I saw a little, old Japanese instructor quietly do this in the Budokan (a massive training arena dedicated to martial arts in the centre of Tokyo) and 300 noisy chattering people instantly stopped and paid attention,

Another thing I've been told on my travels is that the 'shhh' noise is common in all cultures regardless of language. Even remote tribes naturally use this to quieten babies. It's been used since the beginning of time. One theory is that it's the noise that blood makes as it pumps through the body, as heard by the foetus in the womb, I really like that idea. Regardless of the origins there is one thing I do know, the following technique works:

STOP the S.T.O.P. – turning off the little voice with harmony

Think of all your worries and woes. This works really well at night, and I know people that have used this to help with insomnia.

Get comfortable. Take a really deep breath in, pause then breathe out for a long time. Repeat.

Then close your eyes, take a deep breath in and on the exhale make a 'shhh' noise. This could be a series of short 'shhh' or a long 'shhhhhhh' one will feel better than the other, you decide.

After a very short time your mind will quieten.

Now slow the 'shhh' down.

As you do this technique try to think of all the things that bother you. I bet you can't!

The other cool thing is that you should be aware of your muscles relaxing as you do it. Some people find it better if they imagine a loved one doing the 'shhh.'

I love the 'shhh' technique. If you were handed a crying baby or you handed a baby to another responsible human being on this planet, regardless of their race, age, colour, country of origins or language, the chances are the 'shhh' noise would be used to appease the baby. I've already mentioned the power of the 'shhh' to get attention. There is another thing to add to the 'shhh' collection: snakes make a 'shhh' noise too. So what? Well, there is something called the 'snake detection theory' which says that snakes have directly helped man evolve. We have developed heightened senses with regards to danger thanks to the fact that throughout our evolution, even before we were humans, we have lived with the ever present danger from snakes. Why snakes? Because they are pretty unique; the can get anywhere, they are powerful, they are lightning fast, camouflaged, some can kill a human with a bite, some can kill a human by crushing and, scariest of all, some can eat a (small) human whole! So, it's safe to say that they were (and still are) one of the most dangerous creatures we can encounter. If we hear a snake before we see it our hardwired response is to freeze, stop breathing, stop thinking, stop making noise, stop talking until we have defined the location of the little fellow. So, I'm not really sure what actually happens to the brain regarding the 'shhh' technique but I know one thing, the brain goes quiet.

The technique is highly effective with two main types of insomnia:

Onset insomnia – difficulty in falling asleep but sleep ok through the night

Maintenance insomnia – fall asleep ok but wide awake a few hours later

It can also be used at anytime, wherever you are, to stop your S.T.O.P. Pretty powerful right?

CHAPTER 10 : Quietening the mind

Last Word

In my opinion good sleep happens when we are balanced, when we are experiencing homoeostasis. We instinctively know what is bad for us: junk food, illicit drugs, excessive alcohol, smoking, sugar, caffeine, etc. When we feel bad we generally sleep badly.

We also know when our environment is toxic. If we don't feel safe, secure and happy in the space we occupy on this planet then we are in protection rather than growth. In short, we are constantly interpreting our environment as toxic. This is usually caused by a negative relationship with other humans in our proximity but it can be from the disruptive energy from junk and clutter.

It's only been in the last few years that the average person has been able to fill their environment with disruptive and intrusive technology, it's been more recent that the average person could even afford a TV in their bedrooms let alone, tablets, smart phones and voice activated devices. This same technology, although convenient, has actually invaded the sanctuary of our homes with (mainly) negative distractions.

When we have a quality balanced diet our reward is quality balanced slumber. Remember: GIGO – Garbage In Garbage Out or we can CHOOSE QIQO – Quality In Quality Out. The key thing, as you've seen, is that a quality diet needs just a bit of knowledge and research, for example, we need to know that we are not just consuming the right AMOUNT of fruit and veg but the right TYPES. Who knew that magnesium (an important part of our sleep process) has not been as prevalent in our soil for about the last 50 years...about the same time that sleep disruption has become such an issue? So we need to compensate by seeking out food high in magnesium.

Lastly, and most importantly, we need to control what we allow into the profoundly important space we own – our brains. When we download, offload, share, and control our thoughts and worries we are balancing out our minds. We CANNOT do this if we listen to our S.T.O.P. we need to tune into our instincts!

When we balance all aspects of our lives, only then can we expect quality sleep. As I've already said, if we are hydrated, fit and well rested we can deal with ANY situation so much easier. Only then can we acknowledge our ability to cope and it's then that we can develop confidence in ourselves. This all makes a fantastic cocktail for a quality, happy life. Like I say in 'Stress Ninja', when it comes to stress, relationships, friendships, your weight, your fitness, your environment, your thoughts and your life in general, you need to embrace QIQO, because if you do your best to embrace quality there is only one result for your life: quality!

Remember,

You can't have a quality life without

quality sleep!

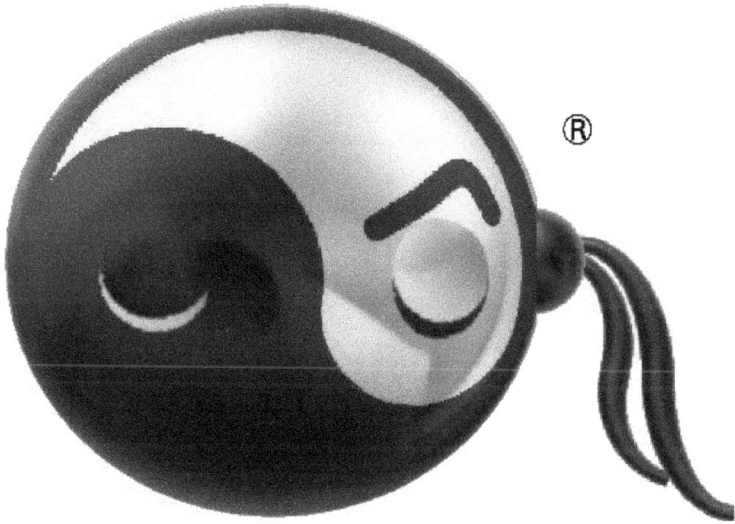

Copyright © Karl Rollison 2019

www.ingramcontent.com/pod-product-compliance
Lightning Source LLC
Chambersburg PA
CBHW072011290326
41934CB00007BA/1056